TETRACYCLINE {BACTERIAL INFECTION}

Dr. Richard A. Gamble

Tetracycline

Tetracycline medication is an anti-microbial used to treat various bacterial contaminations, like urinary lot diseases, skin break out, gonorrhea, chlamydia, and others.

Antibiotic medication is accessible under the accompanying different brand names: Sumycin, Actisite, and Achromycin V.

What Are Measurements of Antibiotic medication?

Measurements of Antibiotic medication:

Container/Tablet

Syrup (on the spur of the moment arranged)

Dose Contemplations - Ought to be given as Follows:

Persistent Bronchitis, Intense Worsening

500 mg orally like clockwork

Skin break out

250-500 mg orally like clockwork

Ehrlichiosis

500 mg orally like clockwork for 7-14 days

Vibrio Cholera

Grown-up: 500 mg orally at regular intervals for 3 days

Pediatric, Single portion: 25 mg/kg orally; not to surpass 1 g/portion

Pediatric, Various portion: 40 mg/kg/day orally isolated at regular intervals for 3 days; not to surpass 2 g/day

Jungle fever, Extreme Treatment (Unlabeled)

Grown-up: 500 mg orally like clockwork for 7 days with quinidine gluconate

Youngsters under 8 years: Not suggested; tooth staining and veneer hypoplasia might happen with use in small kids

Kids north of 8 years: 25-50 mg/kg/day orally partitioned like clockwork, not to surpass 250 mg/portion at regular intervals for 7 days with quinidine gluconate

Measurements Changes

Renal impedance

CrCl 50-80 mL/min: Portion recurrence each 8-12 hours

CrCl 10-50 mL/min: Portion recurrence each 12-24 hours

CrCl under 10 mL/min: Portion recurrence like clockwork

Dosing Contemplations

Acinetobacter spp, Actinomyces israelii, Afipia felis, Bacillus anthracis, Bacteroides spp, Bartonella bacilliformis, Bartonella quintana, Bordetella pertussis, Borrelia recurrentis, Brucella spp, Capnocytophaga canimorsus, Campylobacter jejuni, Chlamydia spp, Citrobacter spp, Coxiella burnetii, Eikenella corrodens, Escherichia coli, Francisella tularensis, Leptospira interrogans, Helicobacter pylori, Klebsiella spp, Listeria monocytogenes, Moraxella catarrhalis, Mycoplasma pneumoniae, Neisseria gonorrhoeae, Propionibacterium acnes, Rickettsiae, Shigella spp, Staphylococcus aureus, Streptococcus pneumoniae, Treponema pallidum, Ureaplasma urealyticum, Vibrio cholerae, Yersinia pestis, Yersinia enterocol tica, Yersinia pseudotuberculosis

General Dosing Rules, pediatric

Youngsters under 8 years: Not suggested; tooth staining and veneer hypoplasia might happen with use in small kids

Kids north of 8 years: 25-50 mg/kg/day orally isolated at regular intervals; not to surpass 3 g/day

Organization

Take while starving; try not to take with dairy items

What Are Secondary effects Related with Utilizing Antibiotic medication?

Normal symptoms of antibiotic medication include:

Staining of teeth and polish hypoplasia (small kids)

The runs

Queasiness

Stomach upset

Loss of craving

White patches or injuries inside your mouth or all the rage

Dark bristly tongue

Inconvenience gulping

Wooziness

Migraine

Bruises or enlarging in your rectal or genital region

Vaginal tingling or release

Stomach cramps

Exfoliative dermatitis

Expanded intracranial strain

Tingling

Loss of craving

Pericarditis

Pigmentation of nails

Spewing

Sumycin (antibiotic medication hydrochloride) is an anti-toxin used to treat a wide range of bacterial diseases, like urinary parcel contaminations, skin break out, gonorrhea, chlamydia, and others. Sumycin is accessible in conventional structure.

What Are Symptoms of Sumycin?

Normal results of Sumycin include:

Sickness, regurgitating, looseness of the bowels, stomach upset, loss of hunger, white patches or bruises inside your mouth or all the rage, enlarged tongue, dark bushy tongue, sore throat, inconvenience gulping, wooziness, cerebral pain, wounds or expanding in your rectal or genital region, or vaginal tingling or release.

Let your primary care physician know if you have serious symptoms of Sumycin including:

Sun related burn (sun responsiveness), nail staining, muscle torment, changes in how much pee, brown or dark tooth staining, deadness or shivering of the hands or feet, strange exhaustion, new indications of disease (e.g., constant sore throat, fever, chills), hearing changes (e.g., ringing in the ears, diminished hearing), simple swelling or dying,serious stomach or stomach torment, yellowing eyes or skin, or dull pee.

Measurements for Sumycin

The standard everyday portion of Sumycin for grown-ups is 500 mg two times/day or 250 mg multiple times/day for gentle to direct contaminations; higher portions might be expected for serious diseases. For kids over eight years old, normal day to day portion of Sumycin is 10 to 20 mg/lb (25 to 50 mg/kg) body weight partitioned in four equivalent dosages.

What Medications, Substances, or Enhancements Associate with Sumycin?

Sumycin might connect with cholesterol-bringing down meds, isotretinoin, tretinoin, acid neutralizers, bismuth subsalicylate (for example Pepto-Bismol), minerals (iron, zinc, calcium, magnesium, and over-the-counter nutrient and mineral enhancements), blood thinners, or penicillin anti-toxins. Let your PCP know all meds you are taking.

Sumycin during Pregnancy or Breastfeeding

Sumycin isn't suggested for use during pregnancy as a result of conceivable damage to a hatchling. Ladies of childbearing age ought to utilize compelling conception prevention while taking this drug. This medicine passes into bosom milk in tiny sums. While there have been no reports of damage to nursing newborn children, counsel your PCP prior to breastfeeding.

Sumycin for oral organization contains antibiotic medication, an anti-toxin secluded from Streptomyces aureofaciens. Antibiotic medication is depicted synthetically as 4-(dimethylamino)- 1, 4, 4a, 5, 5a, 6, 11, 12a-octa-hydro-3, 6, 10, 12, 12a-pentahydroxy-6-methyl-1, 11-dioxo-2-rest thacenecarboxamide; its underlying recipe is:

SUMYCIN (Antibiotic medication Hydrochloride) underlying equation outline

Sumycin '250' and Sumycin '500' Tablets (Antibiotic medication Hydrochloride Tablets) are accessible for oral organization as tablets giving 250 mg and 500 mg antibiotic medication hydrochloride, individually. Dormant fixings: colorants (D&C Red No. 30 Aluminum lake, titanium dioxide), hypromellose, anhydrous lactose, magnesium stearate, microcrystalline cellulose, povidone, pregelatinized starch, stearic corrosive. Likewise, 250 mg contains methylene chloride hydroxypropyl cellulose, triacetin, and 500 mg contains polyethylene glycol, polyparaben, methylparaben, sodium citrate, potassium sorbate, propylparaben, and thickener.

Antibiotic

Antibiotic medications (antibiotic medication, doxycycline, minocycline, tigecycline) are a class of medicine used to oversee and treat different bacterial diseases. Antibiotic medications arrange as protein amalgamation inhibitor anti-toxins and are viewed as expansive range. This movement surveys the signs, activity, and contraindications for antibiotic medications as an important specialist in treating bacterial contaminations. This action will feature the component of activity, unfavorable occasion profile, and applicable collaborations appropriate for individuals from the medical services group associated with patient consideration of these diseases.

These medications can treat rickettsial contaminations, Ehrlichiosis, anaplasmosis, leptospirosis, amebiasis, Actinomycosis, nocardiosis, brucellosis, melioidosis, tularemia, chlamydial contaminations, pelvic provocative infection, syphilis, voyager's loose bowels, early Lyme sickness, skin break out, legionnaire's illness, and Whipple infection. They cover Borrelia recurrentis, Mycobacterium marinum, Mycoplasma pneumoniae, Staphylococcus aureus (counting methicillin-safe S. aureus [MRSA]), Vibrio vulnificus, and vancomycin-safe enterococcus (VRE) (helpless strains). Meningococcal prophylaxis is additionally reachable.

Different signs of antibiotic medications incorporate rosacea, bullous dermatoses, sarcoidosis, Kaposi sarcoma, pyoderma gangrenosum, hidradenitis suppurativa, Sweet condition, a1-antitrypsin lack, panniculitis, pityriasis lichenoides chronica, rheumatoid joint pain, scleroderma, malignant growth, and cardiovascular illnesses (stomach aortic aneurysm and intense myocardial dead tissue).

Instrument of Activity

Protein union is a fundamental necessity of any cell. It includes the utilization of ribosomes, whose occupation is to make an interpretation of a mRNA code into working proteins. In eukaryotes, this happens on ribosomes with the 40S and 60S subunits. In prokaryotes, for example, microorganisms, protein amalgamation happens utilizing ribosomes with the 30S and 50S subunits. At these locales, the ribosome move RNA (tRNA), which is accused of an amino corrosive, ties to the mRNA format. The resulting restricting of every tRNA accused of an amino corrosive adds to the arrangement and lengthening of cell proteins. Antibiotic medications explicitly restrain the 30S ribosomal subunit, blocking the limiting of the aminoacyl-tRNA to the acceptor site on the mRNA-ribosome complex. At the point when this interaction stops, a cell can never again keep up with legitimate working and will not be able to develop or additionally repeat. This sort of debilitation by the antibiotic medications makes them "bacteriostatic."

There is a developing worry over bacterial strains that are impervious to antibiotic medication anti-infection agents. Bacterial qualities that are impervious to antibiotic medications are much of the time encoded on plasmids or adaptable components like transposons. There are two irrefutable components of obstruction, which remember adjustment for ribosomal insurance proteins or efflux siphons. The previous component permits the ribosomes to continue with protein combination no matter what the high intracellular levels of the medication. The last system comprises of different subtypes of transmembrane siphons that drive out solutes, in this example, antimicrobials, out of the cell to forestall cell demise. There is documentation of a third, less concentrated on system of obstruction, which is that of antibiotic medication change. These systems lessen the viability of antibiotic medications, calling for expanded industriousness when clinicians recommend these medications.

Organization

The organization of most antibiotic medications is through the oral course; in any case, skin, intramuscular (IM), and intravenous (IV) types of the medicine do exist. Just oxytetracycline and antibiotic medication organization can be through IM infusion. Oral antibiotic medication assimilation happens fundamentally in the stomach, duodenum, and small digestive tract. They appropriate well in tissues, ascitic liquid, synovial liquid, pleural liquid, and bronchial emissions. Antibiotic medications have unfortunate infiltration into the cerebral spinal liquid. The ingestion of all antibiotic medications diminishes when regulated with multivalent cations like aluminum, calcium, iron, or magnesium. Cations cause chelation of the antibiotic medications, in this way debilitating their retention in the stomach, prompting the discharge of the medication in the pee and excrement.

Antibiotic medications can generally cause GI trouble, including stomach distress, epigastric agony, sickness, spewing, and anorexia. While taking antibiotic medications, staining of teeth and restraint of bone development in kids might happen. A few patients experience photosensitivity, which can appear as a red rash or skin rankling. Photosensitivity responses can be reduced by staying away from direct daylight and tanning hardware or wearing sunscreen and defensive dress when outside.

All the more once in a blue moon, antibiotic medications can cause hepatotoxicity and could compound previous renal disappointment. Further, there have been reports of esophageal ulceration and injuries from antibiotic medication use, which can regularly be tried not to by ingest the medications with satisfactory water and remaining upstanding following utilization. Further, intracranial hypertension (IH, pseudotumor cerebri) associates with antibiotic medication use.

In conclusion, all anti-microbials have suggestions in the advancement of Clostridioides difficile related the runs, including the antibiotic medication class of anti-infection agents.

Contraindications

Antibiotic medications are contraindicated in pregnancy in view of the gamble of hepatotoxicity in the mother, the potential for super durable staining of teeth in the embryo (yellow or brown by all accounts), as well as disability of fetal long bone development. Antibiotic medication use is likewise connected with teeth staining in youngsters younger than eight. Along these lines it ought to be kept away from in pediatric patients under that age.

Clinicians ought to likewise keep away from antibiotic medications in patients with renal disappointment because of the discharge of the medication being principally by the kidneys. In the event that antibiotic medications should be utilized in this gathering of patients, either diminish the measurements as well as increment the stretch between dosages ought to be delayed.

Antibiotic medications really do cross into bosom milk; in this manner, they are protected while breastfeeding. The critical measure of calcium in bosom milk chelates the medication and limits its accessibility to the newborn child.

Checking

The dosing of antibiotic medications is different in grown-ups and kids. Grown-ups may get 1g complete of antibiotic medications every day, which can be separated into 500 mg two times every day or 250 mg four times each day. Higher portions might be given for additional serious contaminations, like 500 mg four times each day. Pediatric patients over eight years of age can get a day to day portion of 25 mg/kg up to 50 mg/kg, isolated into four equivalent dosages.

Ordinary degrees of antibiotic medications accomplished in the serum after oral dosing range from 2 to 5 mcg/ml. Most of antibiotic medications require dosing two to multiple times day to day to keep up with restorative focuses in the serum. All things considered, doxycycline and minocycline have longer end half-lives and license on more than one occasion every day dosing.

Accomplishing satisfactory serum convergences of antibiotic medications might be weakened by stomach settling agents that contain aluminum, calcium, magnesium, iron, zinc, or sodium bicarbonate. In this way, certain food varieties high in these cations, as well as some dairy items, may slow down retention.

Antibiotic medications might deliver oral prophylactic pills less successful. Consequently clinicians ought to emphatically energize the utilization of some type of obstruction assurance in physically dynamic females.

Upgrading Medical care Group Results

Suitably overseeing patients caused with irresistible sicknesses is of most extreme significance to the whole medical care group. As antimicrobial obstruction is on the ascent, guaranteeing the utilization of the legitimate anti-toxin specialist during the destruction of disease is fundamental. The interprofessional medical care group necessities to perceive the significance of designated drug-defenseless treatment. The drug specialist ought to work cooperatively with the prescriber to guarantee that antibiotic medication is the suitable specialist for the disease and confirm dosing and span. This approach will essentially help the patient and give a cultural advantage.

Alongside the clinician and nursing, the drug specialist ought to give patient directing with respect to the prescription. Nursing will be the cutting edge contact for the patient and ought to teach the patient on the most proficient method to take the medication and what signs to look for in accordance with conceivable poisonousness or unfriendly responses. With this interprofessional collaboration, patient results can be enhanced while limiting unfriendly occasions. [Level 5]

The whole local area will benefit and be less in danger of fostering a hazardous medication safe contamination through enough designated treatment of those with irresistible illnesses.

Tetracycline

Antibiotic medication is an anti-infection used to treat a wide range of bacterial contaminations, like urinary plot diseases, skin inflammation, gonorrhea, chlamydia, and others.

Antibiotic medication is accessible under the accompanying different brand names: Sumycin, Actisite, and Achromycin V.

WHAT ARE Doses OF Antibiotic medication?

Measurements of Antibiotic medication:

Case/Tablet

250 mg

500 mg

Syrup (without premeditation arranged)

125mg/5mL

5 mg

Measurement Contemplations - Ought to be given as Follows:

Constant Bronchitis, Intense Worsening

500 mg orally at regular intervals

Skin inflammation

250-500 mg orally at regular intervals

Ehrlichiosis

500 mg orally at regular intervals for 7-14 days

Vibrio Cholera

Grown-up: 500 mg orally at regular intervals for 3 days

Pediatric, Single portion: 25 mg/kg orally; not to surpass 1 g/portion

Pediatric, Various portion: 40 mg/kg/day orally partitioned like clockwork for 3 days; not to surpass 2 g/day

Intestinal sickness, Serious Therapy (Unlabeled)

Grown-up: 500 mg orally like clockwork for 7 days with quinidine gluconate

Youngsters under 8 years: Not suggested; tooth staining and finish hypoplasia might happen with use in small kids

Kids more than 8 years: 25-50 mg/kg/day orally separated at regular intervals, not to surpass 250 mg/portion like clockwork for 7 days with quinidine gluconate

Measurement Alterations

Renal debilitation

CrCl 50-80 mL/min: Portion recurrence each 8-12 hours

CrCl 10-50 mL/min: Portion recurrence each 12-24 hours

CrCl under 10 mL/min: Portion recurrence at regular intervals

Dosing Contemplations

Powerless organic entities

Acinetobacter spp, Actinomyces israelii, Afipia felis, Bacillus anthracis, Bacteroides spp, Bartonella bacilliformis, Bartonella quintana, Bordetella pertussis, Borrelia recurrentis, Brucella spp, Capnocytophaga canimorsus, Campylobacter jejuni, Chlamydia spp, Citrobacter spp, Coxiella burnetii, Eikenella corrodens, Escherichia coli, Francisella tularensis, Leptospira interrogans, Helicobacter pylori, Klebsiella spp, Listeria monocytogenes, Moraxella catarrhalis, Mycoplasma pneumoniae, Neisseria gonorrhoeae, Propionibacterium acnes, Rickettsiae, Shigella spp, Staphylococcus aureus, Streptococcus pneumoniae, Treponema pallidum, Ureaplasma urealyticum, Vibrio cholerae, Yersinia pestis, Yersinia enterocolitica, Yersinia pseudotuberculosis

General Dosing Rules, pediatric

Kids under 8 years: Not suggested; tooth staining and finish hypoplasia might happen with use in small kids

Kids more than 8 years: 25-50 mg/kg/day orally isolated like clockwork; not to surpass 3 g/day

Organization

Take while starving; try not to take with dairy items

WHAT ARE Aftereffects Related WITH Utilizing Antibiotic medication?

Normal results of antibiotic medication include:

Staining of teeth and finish hypoplasia (small kids)

Looseness of the bowels

Sickness

Photosensitivity

Stomach upset

Loss of hunger

White patches or wounds inside your mouth or all the rage

Enlarged tongue

Dark bushy tongue

Sore throat

Inconvenience gulping

Discombobulation

Cerebral pain

Wounds or enlarging in your rectal or genital region

Vaginal tingling or release

More uncommon results of antibiotic medication include:

Stomach cramps

Anti-infection related pseudomembranous colitis

Swelling fontanels in babies

Diabetes insipidus disorder

Esophagitis

Exfoliative dermatitis

Expanded intracranial strain

Tingling

Loss of craving

Pancreatitis

Pericarditis

Pigmentation of nails

Pseudotumor cerebri

Spewing

Serious symptoms of antibiotic medication include:

Burn from the sun (sun awareness)

Muscle torment

Changes in how much pee

Brown or dim tooth staining

Deadness or shivering of the hands or feet

Surprising exhaustion

New indications of contamination (e.g., industrious sore throat, fever, chills)

Hearing changes (e.g., ringing in the ears, diminished hearing)

Simple swelling or dying

Extreme stomach or stomach torment

Yellowing eyes or skin

Dim pee

This is certainly not a total rundown of secondary effects and other serious aftereffects might happen. Call your PCP for data and clinical counsel about incidental effects. You might report aftereffects to FDA at 1-800-FDA-1088.

What different medications interface with antibiotic medication?

On the off chance that your PCP has guided you to involve this prescription for your condition, your primary care physician or drug specialist may currently know about any conceivable medication associations or incidental effects and might be observing you for them. Try not to begin, stop, or change the measurements of this medication or any medication prior to getting additional data from your primary care physician, medical care supplier, or drug specialist first.

Serious Communications of antibiotic medication include:

Acitretin, flibanserin, lomitapide, tretinoin

Antibiotic medication has serious associations with no less than 71 unique medications.

Antibiotic medication has moderate associations with somewhere around 46 unique medications.

Antibiotic medication has gentle communications with something like 26 distinct medications.

This archive doesn't contain every conceivable communication. Hence, prior to utilizing this item, tell your PCP or drug specialist of the multitude of items you use. Keep a rundown of every one of your meds with you, and offer the rundown with your PCP and drug specialist. Check with your doctor assuming you have wellbeing different kinds of feedback.

Admonitions

This drug contains antibiotic medication. Try not to take Sumycin, Actisite, or Achromycin V assuming you are susceptible to antibiotic medication or any fixings contained in this medication.

Keep far away from youngsters. If there should be an occurrence of excess, get clinical assistance or contact a Toxin Control Center right away.

Contraindications

Recorded excessive touchiness

Extreme hepatic brokenness

Impacts of Chronic drug use

No data accessible

Transient Impacts

See "What Are Aftereffects Related with Utilizing Antibiotic medication?"

Long haul Impacts

See "What Are Secondary effects Related with Utilizing Antibiotic medication?"

Alerts

Photosensitivity might happen with delayed openness to daylight or tanning hardware.

Diminish portion in renal impedance.

Consider drug serum level conclusions in delayed treatment.

Antibiotic medication use during tooth advancement (last 50% of pregnancy through age 8 years) can cause long-lasting staining of teeth.

Fanconilike condition might happen with obsolete antibiotic medications.

Intravenous/intramuscular (IV/IM) is presently not industrially accessible.

Pregnancy and Lactation

Utilize foundational antibiotic medication during pregnancy just in Hazardous crises when no more secure medication is free. There is positive proof of human fetal gamble.

Utilize periodontal fiber antibiotic medication with alert during pregnancy on the off chance that the advantages offset the dangers. Creature concentrates on show chance and human investigations are not accessible or neither creature nor human examinations were finished.

Antibiotic medication use during tooth advancement (last 50% of pregnancy through age 8 years) can cause long-lasting staining of teeth.

Antibiotic medication enters bosom milk; a few producers say don't nurture; notwithstanding, the American Foundation of Pediatrics (AAP) considers nursing viable because of calcium chelation of medication and counteraction of its ingestion (long haul security of delayed openness obscure).

Dose Structures and Qualities

Case/tablet

250mg

500mg

Ongoing Bronchitis, Intense Worsening

Regular everyday portion: 500 mg PO q12hr or 250 mg PO q6hr (ie, 1000 mg/day)

Higher portions (eg, 500 mg PO q6hr) might be expected for extreme diseases or for those contaminations which don't answer the more modest dosages

Moderate-to-Serious Skin inflammation

Suggested beginning measurement: 1 g/day PO in partitioned dosages (in light of the judgment of the clinician)

At the point when improvement is noted, step by step decrease portion to support levels going from 125-500 mg/day

A few patients might have the option to keep up with sufficient reduction of injuries with substitute day or irregular treatment

Length of long haul treatment which can securely be suggested has not been laid out

Brucellosis

500 mg PO q6hr for a long time joined by streptomycin, 1 g IM BID for the principal week, then, at that point, qDay the subsequent week

Syphilis

Patients hypersensitive to penicillin

Early syphilis (term <1 year): 500 mg PO q6hr for 15 days

Syphilis (term >1 year [except neurosyphilis]): 500 mg PO q6hr for 30 days

Gonorrhea

Suggested portion: 500 mg PO q6hr for 7 days

Simple urethral, endocervical or rectal contaminations

Contaminations in grown-ups brought about by Chlamydia trachomatis

500 mg PO q6hr for no less than seven days

Different Contaminations

Upper respiratory lot contaminations brought about by Streptococcus pyogenes, Streptococcus pneumoniae and Haemophilus influenzae; antibiotic medication ought not be utilized for streptococcal sickness except if the organic entity has been shown to be vulnerable

Lower respiratory plot diseases brought about by Streptococcus pyogenes, Streptococcus pneumoniae, Mycoplasma pneumoniae (Eaton specialist, and Klebsiella spp)

Skin anc delicate tissue diseases brought about by Streptococcus pyogenes, Staphylococcus aureus; antibiotic medications are not the medications of decision in that frame of mind of a staphylococcal contaminations

Contaminations brought about by rickettsia including Rough Mountain spotted fever, typhus bunch diseases, Q fever, rickettsialpox

Psittacosis brought about by Chlamydophila psittaci

Contaminations brought about by Chlamydia trachomatis (eg, simple urethral, endocervical or rectal diseases, incorporation conjunctivitis, trachoma, and lymphogranuloma venereum)

Granuloma inguinale brought about by Klebsiella granulomatis Backsliding fever brought about by Borrelia spp Bartonellosis brought about by Bartonella bacilliformis

Chancroid brought about by haemophilus ducreyi

Tularemia brought about by Francisella tularensis

Plaque brought about by Yersinia pestis

Cholera brought about by Vibrio cholerae

Brucellosis brought about by Brucella species (antibiotic medication might be utilized related to an aminoglycoside)

Contaminations because of Campylobacter hatchling

As adjunctive treatment in gastrointestinal amebiasis brought about by Entamoeba histolytica

Urinary plot diseases brought about by defenseless strains (eg, Escherichia coli, Klebsiella)

Different contaminations brought about by helpless gram-negative organic entities, for example, E coli, Enterobacter aerogenes, Shigella spp, Acinetobacter spp, Klebsiella spp, and Bacteroides spp

In serious skin break out, adjunctive treatment with antibiotic medication might be valuable

Different Contaminations (Penicillin-Safe)

Syphilis and yaws brought about by Treponema pallidum and pertenue, individually

Vincent's contamination brought about by Fusobacterium fusiforme

Diseases brought about by Neisseria gonorrhoeae

Bacillus anthracis made by Bacillus anthracis

Contaminations due Listeria monocytogenes

Actinomycosis brought about by Actinomyces spp

Diseases because of Clostridium spp

Measurement Changes

Renal disability

Complete measurements ought to be diminished by decrease of suggested individual dosages and additionally by broadening time spans between portions

Dosing Contemplations

In the treatment of streptococcal contaminations, directed for something like 10 days

Similarly as with different antibacterials, utilization of this medication might bring about excess of nonsusceptible creatures, including parasites

Assuming superinfection happens, end antibacterial and foundation proper treatment

Treat all contaminations because of Gathering A beta-hemolytic streptococci for something like 10 days

Perform entry point and waste or other surgeries related to antibacterial treatment, when demonstrated

Recommending antibiotic medication without a trace of demonstrated or emphatically thought bacterial disease or a prophylactic sign is probably not going to give advantage to the patient and expands the gamble of the improvement of medication safe microbes

microbes, particular bacterium, any of a gathering of minuscule single-celled organic entities that live in huge numbers in pretty much every climate on The planet, from remote ocean vents to far beneath Earth's surface to the gastrointestinal systems of people.

Microscopic organisms come up short on film bound core and other inward designs and are consequently positioned among the unicellular living things called prokaryotes. Prokaryotes are the prevailing living animals on the planet, having been available for maybe 3/4 of Earth history and having adjusted to practically all suitable natural environments. Collectively, they show extremely different metabolic capacities and can utilize practically any natural compound, and a few inorganic mixtures, as a food source. A few microorganisms can cause illnesses in people, creatures, or plants, yet most are innocuous and are useful natural specialists whose metabolic exercises support higher living things. Different microorganisms are symbionts of plants and spineless creatures, where they complete significant capabilities for the host, like nitrogen obsession and cellulose corruption. Without prokaryotes, soil wouldn't be ripe, and dead natural material would rot considerably more leisurely. A few microscopic organisms are broadly utilized in the planning of food sources, synthetics, and anti-microbials. Investigations of the connections between various gatherings of microscopic organisms keep on yielding new experiences into the beginning of life on the planet and instruments of development.

The bacterial cell

Microbes as prokaryotes

All living creatures on Earth are comprised of one of two fundamental sorts of cells: eukaryotic cells, in which the hereditary material is encased inside an atomic layer, or prokaryotic cells, in which the hereditary material isn't isolated from the remainder of the cell. Generally, all prokaryotic cells were called microbes and were ordered in the prokaryotic realm Monera. Be that as it may, their characterization as Monera, comparable in scientific categorization to different realms — Plantae, Animalia, Growths, and Protista — downplayed the noteworthy hereditary and metabolic variety showed by prokaryotic cells comparative with eukaryotic cells. In the last part of the 1970s American microbiologist Carl Woese spearheaded a significant change in characterization by putting all organic entities into three spaces — Eukarya, Microorganisms (initially called Eubacteria), and Archaea (initially called Archaebacteria) — to mirror the three old lines of development. The prokaryotic living beings that were previously known as microscopic organisms were then partitioned into two of these spaces, Microbes and Archaea. Microscopic organisms and Archaea are hastily comparative; for instance, they don't have intracellular organelles, and they have round DNA. Notwithstanding, they are in a general sense unmistakable, and their partition depends on the hereditary proof for their old and separate transformative genealogies, as well as essential contrasts in their science and physiology. Individuals from these two prokaryotic spaces are as not the same as each other as they are from eukaryotic cells.

Prokaryotic cells (i.e., Microorganisms and Archaea) are generally not the same as the eukaryotic cells that comprise different types of life. Prokaryotic cells are characterized by a lot more straightforward plan than is tracked down in eukaryotic cells. The most-clear disentanglement is the absence of intracellular organelles, which are highlights normal for eukaryotic cells. Organelles are discrete film encased structures that are contained in the cytoplasm and incorporate the core, where hereditary data is held, replicated, and communicated; the mitochondria and chloroplasts, where substance or light energy is changed over into metabolic energy; the lysosome, where ingested proteins are processed and different supplements are made accessible; furthermore, the endoplasmic reticulum and the Golgi device, where the proteins that are blended by and set free from the cell are gathered, changed, and traded. Each of the exercises performed by organelles additionally occur in microorganisms, yet they are not done by specific designs. Furthermore, prokaryotic cells are generally a lot more modest than eukaryotic cells. The little size, basic plan, and expansive metabolic abilities of microorganisms permit them to develop and separate quickly and to occupy and prosper in practically any climate.

Prokaryotic and eukaryotic cells contrast in numerous alternate ways, including lipid arrangement, construction of key metabolic catalysts, reactions to anti-toxins and poisons, and the system of articulation of hereditary data. Eukaryotic organic entities contain various straight chromosomes with qualities that are a lot bigger than they should be to encode the union of proteins. Significant parts of the ribonucleic corrosive (RNA) duplicate of the hereditary data (deoxyribonucleic corrosive, or DNA) are disposed of, and the leftover courier RNA (mRNA) is considerably adjusted before it is converted into protein. Conversely, microscopic organisms have one round chromosome that contains their hereditary data, and their mRNAs are all precise duplicates of their qualities and are not adjusted.

Variety of design of microorganisms

Albeit bacterial cells are a lot more modest and less difficult in structure than eukaryotic cells, the microorganisms are an extremely different gathering of creatures that vary in size, shape, territory, and digestion. A large part of the information about microscopic organisms has come from investigations of sickness causing microorganisms, which are all the more promptly secluded in unadulterated culture and more effortlessly researched than are a considerable lot of the free-living types of microbes. It should be noticed that some free-living microbes are very unique in relation to the microorganisms that are adjusted to live as creature parasites or symbionts. Along these lines, there are no outright guidelines about bacterial arrangement or construction, and there are numerous exemptions for any broad assertion.

Individual microorganisms can accept one of three fundamental shapes: circular (coccus), rodlike (bacillus), or bended (vibrio, spirillum, or spirochete). Impressive variety is found in the genuine states of microbes, and cells can be extended or packed in one aspect. Microscopic organisms that don't separate from each other after cell division structure trademark groups that are useful in their recognizable proof. For instance, a few cocci are found for the most part two by two, including Streptococcus pneumoniae, a pneumococcus that causes bacterial lobar pneumonia, and Neisseria gonorrhoeae, a gonococcus that causes the physically communicated sickness gonorrhea. Most streptococci look like a long strand of dots, though the staphylococci structure irregular bunches (the name "staphylococci" is gotten from the Greek word staphyle, signifying "group of grapes"). Moreover, a few coccal microorganisms happen as square or cubical parcels. The bar molded bacilli for the most part happen independently, however a few strains structure long chains, for example, poles of the corynebacteria, typical occupants of the mouth that are habitually connected to each other indiscriminately points. A few bacilli have pointed closes, though others have squared finishes, and a few poles are bowed into a comma shape. These bowed bars are in many cases called vibrios and incorporate Vibrio cholerae, which causes cholera. Different states of microbes incorporate the spirilla, which are bowed and rebent, and the spirochetes, which structure a helix like a wine tool, in which the phone body is folded over a focal fiber called the pivotal fiber.

Microscopic organisms are the littlest living substances. A normal size bacterium —, for example, the bar molded Escherichia coli, an ordinary occupant of the digestive system of people and creatures — is around 2 micrometers (μm; millionths of a meter) long and 0.5 μm in measurement, and the round cells of Staphylococcus aureus ultimately depend on 1 μm in breadth. A couple of bacterial sorts are significantly more modest, for example, Mycoplasma pneumoniae, which is perhaps of the littlest bacterium, going from around 0.1 to 0.25 μm in width and around 1 to 1.5 μm long; the bar molded Bordetella pertussis, which is the causative specialist of beating hack, going from

0.2 to 0.5 µm in distance across and 0.5 to 1 µm long; what's more, the wine tool formed Treponema pallidum, which is the causative specialist of syphilis, averaging simply 0.1 to 0.2 µm in breadth however 6 to 15 µm long. The cyanobacterium Synechococcus midpoints around 0.5 to 1.6 µm in breadth.

A few microorganisms are moderately enormous, for example, Azotobacter, which has breadths of 2 to 5 µm or more; what's more, Achromatium, which has a base width of 5 µm and a most extreme length of 100 µm, contingent upon the species. Goliath microorganisms can be apparent with the independent eye, for example, Thiomargarita namibiensis, which midpoints 750 µm in breadth; T. magnifica, which midpoints 700 µm in breadth and 1 cm long; furthermore, the bar formed Epulopiscium fishelsoni, which goes from 30 to more than 600 µm long.

Microbes are unicellular microorganisms and accordingly are by and large not coordinated into tissues. Every bacterium develops and partitions autonomously of some other bacterium, despite the fact that totals of microscopic organisms, in some cases containing individuals from various species, are habitually found. Numerous microorganisms can shape totaled structures called biofilms. Living beings in biofilms frequently show considerably various properties from a similar creature in the singular state or the planktonic state. Microorganisms that have accumulated into biofilms can convey data about populace size and metabolic state. This kind of correspondence is called majority detecting and works by the creation of little atoms called autoinducers or pheromones. The centralization of majority detecting particles — most usually peptides or acylated homoserine lactones (AHLs; exceptional flagging synthetics) — is connected with the quantity of microorganisms of the equivalent or various species that are in the biofilm and helps coordinate the way of behaving of the biofilm.

Morphological highlights of microorganisms

The Gram stain

Microorganisms are little to such an extent that their presence was just first perceived in 1677, when the Dutch naturalist Antonie van Leeuwenhoek saw minuscule creatures in different substances with the guide of crude magnifying lens (more comparative in plan to current amplifying glasses than present day magnifying lens), some of which were able to do more than 200-overlap amplification. Presently microbes are generally inspected under light magnifying instruments able to do more than 1,000-crease amplification; notwithstanding, subtleties of their inward construction can be noticed exclusively with the guide of considerably more impressive transmission electron magnifying instruments. Except if unique stage contrast magnifying instruments are utilized, microorganisms must be stained with a shaded color so they will stand apart from their experience.

One of the most helpful staining responses for microscopic organisms is known as the Gram stain, created in 1884 by the Danish doctor Hans Christian Gram. Microscopic organisms in suspension are fixed to a glass slide by brief warming and afterward presented to two colors that consolidate to shape an enormous blue color complex inside every cell. At the point when the slide is flushed with a liquor arrangement, gram-positive microbes hold the blue tone and gram-negative microscopic organisms lose the blue tone. The slide is then stained with a more fragile pink color that makes the gram-negative microscopic organisms become pink, though the gram-positive microbes stay blue. The Gram stain responds to contrasts in the construction of the bacterial cell surface, contrasts that are evident when the cells are seen under an electron magnifying lens.

The cell envelope

The bacterial cell surface (or envelope) can change extensively in its construction, and it assumes a focal part in the properties and capacities of the cell. The one element present in all cells is the cytoplasmic film, what isolates within the cell from its outside climate, controls the progression of supplements, keeps up with the appropriate intracellular milieu, and forestalls the deficiency of the cell's items. The cytoplasmic film does numerous essential cell capabilities, including energy age, protein emission, chromosome isolation, and productive dynamic vehicle of supplements. It is a common unit layer made out of proteins and lipids, essentially like the film that encompasses every single eukaryotic cell. It shows up in electron micrographs as a triple-layered construction of lipids and proteins that totally encompass the cytoplasm.

Lying beyond this layer is an inflexible wall that decides the state of the bacterial cell. The wall is made of a colossal particle called peptidoglycan (or murein). In gram-positive microbes the peptidoglycan structures a thick meshlike layer that holds the blue color of the Gram stain by catching it in the cell. Conversely, in gram-negative microorganisms the peptidoglycan layer is exceptionally slim (only a couple of particles profound), and the blue color is effortlessly cleaned out of the cell.

Peptidoglycan happens just in the Microorganisms (with the exception of those without a cell wall, like Mycoplasma). Peptidoglycan is a long-chain polymer of two rehashing sugars (N-acetylglucosamine and N-acetyl muramic corrosive), in which contiguous sugar binds are connected to each other by peptide spans that present unbending security. The idea of the peptide spans contrasts extensively between types of microscopic organisms yet in everyday comprises of four amino acids: L-alanine connected to D-glutamic corrosive, connected to either diaminopimelic corrosive in gram-negative microbes or L-lysine, L-ornithine, or diaminopimelic corrosive in gram-positive microorganisms, which is at long last connected to D-alanine. In gram-negative microorganisms the peptide spans associate the D-alanine on one chain to the diaminopimelic corrosive on another chain. In gram-positive microscopic organisms there can be an extra peptide chain that broadens the scope of the cross-connect; for instance, there is an extra scaffold of five glycines in Staphylococcus aureus.

Peptidoglycan amalgamation is the objective of numerous valuable antimicrobial specialists, including the β-lactam anti-toxins (e.g., penicillin) that block the cross-connecting of the peptide spans. A portion of the proteins that creatures incorporate as normal antibacterial safeguard factors assault the cell walls of microbes. For instance, a catalyst called lysozyme parts the sugar chains that are the foundation of peptidoglycan atoms. The activity of any of these specialists debilitates the cell wall and upsets the bacterium.